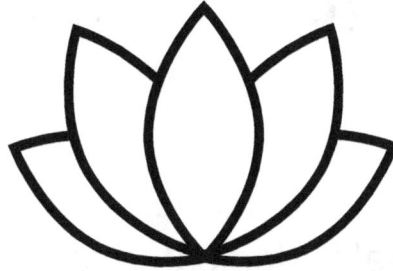

THIS BOOK BELONGS TO:

CONTACT INFORMATION	
NAME	
ADDRESS	
PHONE #	
EMAIL	

DEDICATION

This Meditation Journal is dedicated to all the people who want to keep track of their meditation and mindfulness journey.

You are my inspiration for producing this book and I'm honored to be a part of your record-keeping and organization.

HOW TO USE THIS BOOK

This guided Meditation Journal will help you by accurately recording daily meditations, self-care goals, and reflections in an easy to use format.

Here are examples of information for you to fill in and write the details of your book.

Fill in the following information:

1. Date, Time, and Length - Log day, time, and length of your meditation session.

2. Mood Tracker - Checklist for how you felt before and after meditation (good, neutral, stressed).

3. Thoughts/Notes - Write your thoughts and feelings during the meditation session.

4. Sleep Tracker - Record sleep quality, sleep hours, bedtime, and dream notes.

5. Self Care Tracker - Record activities for your mind, spirit, exercise, and physical activities.

6. Mindfulness - Jot down positive affirmations and gratitude.

7. Meditation Tracker Pages - Color one image for each day of your meditation sessions.

MEDITATION LOG

DATE		TIME		HOW LONG	

MOOD TRACKER

BEFORE	AFTER	THOUGHTS / NOTES ON YOUR MEDITATION
□ GOOD	□ GOOD	
□ NEUTRAL	□ NEUTRAL	
□ STRESSED	□ STRESSED	

SLEEP TRACKER

SLEEP QUALITY	HOW MANY HOURS DID YOU SLEEP?	DREAM NOTES
□ GOOD		
□ NEUTRAL	WHAT TIME DID YOU GO TO BED?	
□ STRESSED	□ AM □ PM	

SELF CARE TRACKER

MIND / SPIRIT	EXERCISE / PHYSICAL ACTIVITY

MINDFULNESS

POSITIVE AFFIRMATIONS	GRATITUDE

MEDITATION LOG

DATE		TIME		HOW LONG	

MOOD TRACKER

BEFORE	AFTER	THOUGHTS / NOTES ON YOUR MEDITATION
□ GOOD	□ GOOD	
□ NEUTRAL	□ NEUTRAL	
□ STRESSED	□ STRESSED	

SLEEP TRACKER

SLEEP QUALITY	HOW MANY HOURS DID YOU SLEEP?	DREAM NOTES
□ GOOD		
□ NEUTRAL	WHAT TIME DID YOU GO TO BED?	
□ STRESSED	□ AM □ PM	

SELF CARE TRACKER

MIND / SPIRIT	EXERCISE / PHYSICAL ACTIVITY

MINDFULNESS

POSITIVE AFFIRMATIONS	GRATITUDE

MEDITATION LOG

DATE		TIME		HOW LONG	

MOOD TRACKER

BEFORE	AFTER	THOUGHTS / NOTES ON YOUR MEDITATION
□ GOOD	□ GOOD	
□ NEUTRAL	□ NEUTRAL	
□ STRESSED	□ STRESSED	

SLEEP TRACKER

SLEEP QUALITY	HOW MANY HOURS DID YOU SLEEP?	DREAM NOTES
□ GOOD		
□ NEUTRAL	WHAT TIME DID YOU GO TO BED?	
□ STRESSED	□ AM □ PM	

SELF CARE TRACKER

MIND / SPIRIT	EXERCISE / PHYSICAL ACTIVITY

MINDFULNESS

POSITIVE AFFIRMATIONS	GRATITUDE

MEDITATION LOG

DATE		TIME		HOW LONG	

MOOD TRACKER

BEFORE	AFTER	THOUGHTS / NOTES ON YOUR MEDITATION
□ GOOD	□ GOOD	
□ NEUTRAL	□ NEUTRAL	
□ STRESSED	□ STRESSED	

SLEEP TRACKER

SLEEP QUALITY	HOW MANY HOURS DID YOU SLEEP?	DREAM NOTES
□ GOOD		
□ NEUTRAL	WHAT TIME DID YOU GO TO BED?	
□ STRESSED	□ AM □ PM	

SELF CARE TRACKER

MIND / SPIRIT	EXERCISE / PHYSICAL ACTIVITY

MINDFULNESS

POSITIVE AFFIRMATIONS	GRATITUDE

MEDITATION LOG

DATE		TIME		HOW LONG	

MOOD TRACKER

BEFORE	AFTER	THOUGHTS / NOTES ON YOUR MEDITATION
□ GOOD	□ GOOD	
□ NEUTRAL	□ NEUTRAL	
□ STRESSED	□ STRESSED	

SLEEP TRACKER

SLEEP QUALITY	HOW MANY HOURS DID YOU SLEEP?	DREAM NOTES
□ GOOD		
□ NEUTRAL	WHAT TIME DID YOU GO TO BED?	
□ STRESSED	□ AM □ PM	

SELF CARE TRACKER

MIND / SPIRIT	EXERCISE / PHYSICAL ACTIVITY

MINDFULNESS

POSITIVE AFFIRMATIONS	GRATITUDE

MEDITATION LOG

DATE		TIME		HOW LONG	

MOOD TRACKER

BEFORE	AFTER	THOUGHTS / NOTES ON YOUR MEDITATION
□ GOOD	□ GOOD	
□ NEUTRAL	□ NEUTRAL	
□ STRESSED	□ STRESSED	

SLEEP TRACKER

SLEEP QUALITY	HOW MANY HOURS DID YOU SLEEP?	DREAM NOTES
□ GOOD		
□ NEUTRAL	**WHAT TIME DID YOU GO TO BED?**	
□ STRESSED	□ AM □ PM	

SELF CARE TRACKER

MIND / SPIRIT	EXERCISE / PHYSICAL ACTIVITY

MINDFULNESS

POSITIVE AFFIRMATIONS	GRATITUDE

MEDITATION LOG

DATE		TIME		HOW LONG	

MOOD TRACKER

BEFORE	AFTER	THOUGHTS / NOTES ON YOUR MEDITATION
□ GOOD	□ GOOD	
□ NEUTRAL	□ NEUTRAL	
□ STRESSED	□ STRESSED	

SLEEP TRACKER

SLEEP QUALITY	HOW MANY HOURS DID YOU SLEEP?	DREAM NOTES
□ GOOD		
□ NEUTRAL	WHAT TIME DID YOU GO TO BED?	
□ STRESSED	□ AM □ PM	

SELF CARE TRACKER

MIND / SPIRIT	EXERCISE / PHYSICAL ACTIVITY

MINDFULNESS

POSITIVE AFFIRMATIONS	GRATITUDE

MEDITATION LOG

DATE		TIME		HOW LONG	

MOOD TRACKER

BEFORE	AFTER	THOUGHTS / NOTES ON YOUR MEDITATION
□ GOOD	□ GOOD	
□ NEUTRAL	□ NEUTRAL	
□ STRESSED	□ STRESSED	

SLEEP TRACKER

SLEEP QUALITY	HOW MANY HOURS DID YOU SLEEP?	DREAM NOTES
□ GOOD		
□ NEUTRAL	WHAT TIME DID YOU GO TO BED?	
□ STRESSED	□ AM □ PM	

SELF CARE TRACKER

MIND / SPIRIT	EXERCISE / PHYSICAL ACTIVITY

MINDFULNESS

POSITIVE AFFIRMATIONS	GRATITUDE

MEDITATION LOG

DATE		TIME		HOW LONG	

MOOD TRACKER

BEFORE	AFTER	THOUGHTS / NOTES ON YOUR MEDITATION
□ GOOD	□ GOOD	
□ NEUTRAL	□ NEUTRAL	
□ STRESSED	□ STRESSED	

SLEEP TRACKER

SLEEP QUALITY	HOW MANY HOURS DID YOU SLEEP?	DREAM NOTES
□ GOOD		
□ NEUTRAL	WHAT TIME DID YOU GO TO BED?	
□ STRESSED	□ AM □ PM	

SELF CARE TRACKER

MIND / SPIRIT	EXERCISE / PHYSICAL ACTIVITY

MINDFULNESS

POSITIVE AFFIRMATIONS	GRATITUDE

MEDITATION LOG

DATE		TIME		HOW LONG	

MOOD TRACKER

BEFORE	AFTER	THOUGHTS / NOTES ON YOUR MEDITATION
□ GOOD	□ GOOD	
□ NEUTRAL	□ NEUTRAL	
□ STRESSED	□ STRESSED	

SLEEP TRACKER

SLEEP QUALITY	HOW MANY HOURS DID YOU SLEEP?	DREAM NOTES
□ GOOD		
□ NEUTRAL	WHAT TIME DID YOU GO TO BED?	
□ STRESSED	□ AM □ PM	

SELF CARE TRACKER

MIND / SPIRIT	EXERCISE / PHYSICAL ACTIVITY

MINDFULNESS

POSITIVE AFFIRMATIONS	GRATITUDE

MEDITATION LOG

DATE		TIME		HOW LONG	

MOOD TRACKER

BEFORE	AFTER	THOUGHTS / NOTES ON YOUR MEDITATION
□ GOOD	□ GOOD	
□ NEUTRAL	□ NEUTRAL	
□ STRESSED	□ STRESSED	

SLEEP TRACKER

SLEEP QUALITY	HOW MANY HOURS DID YOU SLEEP?	DREAM NOTES
□ GOOD		
□ NEUTRAL	WHAT TIME DID YOU GO TO BED?	
□ STRESSED	□ AM □ PM	

SELF CARE TRACKER

MIND / SPIRIT	EXERCISE / PHYSICAL ACTIVITY

MINDFULNESS

POSITIVE AFFIRMATIONS	GRATITUDE

MEDITATION LOG

DATE		TIME		HOW LONG	

MOOD TRACKER

BEFORE	AFTER	THOUGHTS / NOTES ON YOUR MEDITATION
□ GOOD	□ GOOD	
□ NEUTRAL	□ NEUTRAL	
□ STRESSED	□ STRESSED	

SLEEP TRACKER

SLEEP QUALITY	HOW MANY HOURS DID YOU SLEEP?	DREAM NOTES
□ GOOD		
□ NEUTRAL	WHAT TIME DID YOU GO TO BED?	
□ STRESSED	□ AM □ PM	

SELF CARE TRACKER

MIND / SPIRIT	EXERCISE / PHYSICAL ACTIVITY

MINDFULNESS

POSITIVE AFFIRMATIONS	GRATITUDE

MEDITATION LOG

DATE		TIME		HOW LONG	

MOOD TRACKER

BEFORE	AFTER	THOUGHTS / NOTES ON YOUR MEDITATION
□ GOOD	□ GOOD	
□ NEUTRAL	□ NEUTRAL	
□ STRESSED	□ STRESSED	

SLEEP TRACKER

SLEEP QUALITY	HOW MANY HOURS DID YOU SLEEP?	DREAM NOTES
□ GOOD		
□ NEUTRAL	**WHAT TIME DID YOU GO TO BED?**	
□ STRESSED	□ AM □ PM	

SELF CARE TRACKER

MIND / SPIRIT	EXERCISE / PHYSICAL ACTIVITY

MINDFULNESS

POSITIVE AFFIRMATIONS	GRATITUDE

MEDITATION LOG

DATE		TIME		HOW LONG	

MOOD TRACKER

BEFORE	AFTER	THOUGHTS / NOTES ON YOUR MEDITATION
□ GOOD	□ GOOD	
□ NEUTRAL	□ NEUTRAL	
□ STRESSED	□ STRESSED	

SLEEP TRACKER

SLEEP QUALITY	HOW MANY HOURS DID YOU SLEEP?	DREAM NOTES
□ GOOD		
□ NEUTRAL	**WHAT TIME DID YOU GO TO BED?**	
□ STRESSED	□ AM □ PM	

SELF CARE TRACKER

MIND / SPIRIT	EXERCISE / PHYSICAL ACTIVITY

MINDFULNESS

POSITIVE AFFIRMATIONS	GRATITUDE

MEDITATION LOG

DATE			TIME		HOW LONG	

MOOD TRACKER

BEFORE	AFTER	THOUGHTS / NOTES ON YOUR MEDITATION
□ GOOD	□ GOOD	
□ NEUTRAL	□ NEUTRAL	
□ STRESSED	□ STRESSED	

SLEEP TRACKER

SLEEP QUALITY	HOW MANY HOURS DID YOU SLEEP?	DREAM NOTES
□ GOOD		
□ NEUTRAL	WHAT TIME DID YOU GO TO BED?	
□ STRESSED	□ AM □ PM	

SELF CARE TRACKER

MIND / SPIRIT	EXERCISE / PHYSICAL ACTIVITY

MINDFULNESS

POSITIVE AFFIRMATIONS	GRATITUDE

MEDITATION LOG

DATE		TIME		HOW LONG	

MOOD TRACKER

BEFORE	AFTER	THOUGHTS / NOTES ON YOUR MEDITATION
□ GOOD	□ GOOD	
□ NEUTRAL	□ NEUTRAL	
□ STRESSED	□ STRESSED	

SLEEP TRACKER

SLEEP QUALITY	HOW MANY HOURS DID YOU SLEEP?	DREAM NOTES
□ GOOD		
□ NEUTRAL	**WHAT TIME DID YOU GO TO BED?**	
□ STRESSED	□ AM □ PM	

SELF CARE TRACKER

MIND / SPIRIT	EXERCISE / PHYSICAL ACTIVITY

MINDFULNESS

POSITIVE AFFIRMATIONS	GRATITUDE

MEDITATION LOG

DATE		TIME		HOW LONG	

MOOD TRACKER

BEFORE	AFTER	THOUGHTS / NOTES ON YOUR MEDITATION
□ GOOD	□ GOOD	
□ NEUTRAL	□ NEUTRAL	
□ STRESSED	□ STRESSED	

SLEEP TRACKER

SLEEP QUALITY	HOW MANY HOURS DID YOU SLEEP?	DREAM NOTES
□ GOOD		
□ NEUTRAL	WHAT TIME DID YOU GO TO BED?	
□ STRESSED	□ AM □ PM	

SELF CARE TRACKER

MIND / SPIRIT	EXERCISE / PHYSICAL ACTIVITY

MINDFULNESS

POSITIVE AFFIRMATIONS	GRATITUDE

MEDITATION LOG

DATE		TIME		HOW LONG	

MOOD TRACKER

BEFORE	AFTER	THOUGHTS / NOTES ON YOUR MEDITATION
□ GOOD	□ GOOD	
□ NEUTRAL	□ NEUTRAL	
□ STRESSED	□ STRESSED	

SLEEP TRACKER

SLEEP QUALITY	HOW MANY HOURS DID YOU SLEEP?	DREAM NOTES
□ GOOD		
□ NEUTRAL	WHAT TIME DID YOU GO TO BED?	
□ STRESSED	□ AM □ PM	

SELF CARE TRACKER

MIND / SPIRIT	EXERCISE / PHYSICAL ACTIVITY

MINDFULNESS

POSITIVE AFFIRMATIONS	GRATITUDE

MEDITATION LOG

DATE		TIME		HOW LONG	

MOOD TRACKER

BEFORE	AFTER	THOUGHTS / NOTES ON YOUR MEDITATION
□ GOOD	□ GOOD	
□ NEUTRAL	□ NEUTRAL	
□ STRESSED	□ STRESSED	

SLEEP TRACKER

SLEEP QUALITY	HOW MANY HOURS DID YOU SLEEP?	DREAM NOTES
□ GOOD		
□ NEUTRAL	WHAT TIME DID YOU GO TO BED?	
□ STRESSED	□ AM □ PM	

SELF CARE TRACKER

MIND / SPIRIT	EXERCISE / PHYSICAL ACTIVITY

MINDFULNESS

POSITIVE AFFIRMATIONS	GRATITUDE

MEDITATION LOG

DATE		TIME		HOW LONG	

MOOD TRACKER

BEFORE	AFTER	THOUGHTS / NOTES ON YOUR MEDITATION
□ GOOD	□ GOOD	
□ NEUTRAL	□ NEUTRAL	
□ STRESSED	□ STRESSED	

SLEEP TRACKER

SLEEP QUALITY	HOW MANY HOURS DID YOU SLEEP?	DREAM NOTES
□ GOOD		
□ NEUTRAL	WHAT TIME DID YOU GO TO BED?	
□ STRESSED	□ AM □ PM	

SELF CARE TRACKER

MIND / SPIRIT	EXERCISE / PHYSICAL ACTIVITY

MINDFULNESS

POSITIVE AFFIRMATIONS	GRATITUDE

MEDITATION LOG

DATE		TIME		HOW LONG	

MOOD TRACKER

BEFORE	AFTER	THOUGHTS / NOTES ON YOUR MEDITATION
□ GOOD	□ GOOD	
□ NEUTRAL	□ NEUTRAL	
□ STRESSED	□ STRESSED	

SLEEP TRACKER

SLEEP QUALITY	HOW MANY HOURS DID YOU SLEEP?	DREAM NOTES
□ GOOD		
□ NEUTRAL	**WHAT TIME DID YOU GO TO BED?**	
□ STRESSED	□ AM □ PM	

SELF CARE TRACKER

MIND / SPIRIT	EXERCISE / PHYSICAL ACTIVITY

MINDFULNESS

POSITIVE AFFIRMATIONS	GRATITUDE

MEDITATION LOG

DATE		TIME		HOW LONG	

MOOD TRACKER

BEFORE	AFTER	THOUGHTS / NOTES ON YOUR MEDITATION
□ GOOD	□ GOOD	
□ NEUTRAL	□ NEUTRAL	
□ STRESSED	□ STRESSED	

SLEEP TRACKER

SLEEP QUALITY	HOW MANY HOURS DID YOU SLEEP?	DREAM NOTES
□ GOOD		
□ NEUTRAL	WHAT TIME DID YOU GO TO BED?	
□ STRESSED	□ AM □ PM	

SELF CARE TRACKER

MIND / SPIRIT	EXERCISE / PHYSICAL ACTIVITY

MINDFULNESS

POSITIVE AFFIRMATIONS	GRATITUDE

MEDITATION LOG

DATE		TIME		HOW LONG	

MOOD TRACKER

BEFORE	AFTER	THOUGHTS / NOTES ON YOUR MEDITATION
□ GOOD	□ GOOD	
□ NEUTRAL	□ NEUTRAL	
□ STRESSED	□ STRESSED	

SLEEP TRACKER

SLEEP QUALITY	HOW MANY HOURS DID YOU SLEEP?	DREAM NOTES
□ GOOD		
□ NEUTRAL	WHAT TIME DID YOU GO TO BED?	
□ STRESSED	□ AM □ PM	

SELF CARE TRACKER

MIND / SPIRIT	EXERCISE / PHYSICAL ACTIVITY

MINDFULNESS

POSITIVE AFFIRMATIONS	GRATITUDE

MEDITATION LOG

DATE		TIME		HOW LONG	

MOOD TRACKER

BEFORE	AFTER	THOUGHTS / NOTES ON YOUR MEDITATION
□ GOOD	□ GOOD	
□ NEUTRAL	□ NEUTRAL	
□ STRESSED	□ STRESSED	

SLEEP TRACKER

SLEEP QUALITY	HOW MANY HOURS DID YOU SLEEP?	DREAM NOTES
□ GOOD		
□ NEUTRAL	WHAT TIME DID YOU GO TO BED?	
□ STRESSED	□ AM □ PM	

SELF CARE TRACKER

MIND / SPIRIT	EXERCISE / PHYSICAL ACTIVITY

MINDFULNESS

POSITIVE AFFIRMATIONS	GRATITUDE

MEDITATION LOG

DATE		TIME		HOW LONG	

MOOD TRACKER

BEFORE	AFTER	THOUGHTS / NOTES ON YOUR MEDITATION
□ GOOD	□ GOOD	
□ NEUTRAL	□ NEUTRAL	
□ STRESSED	□ STRESSED	

SLEEP TRACKER

SLEEP QUALITY	HOW MANY HOURS DID YOU SLEEP?	DREAM NOTES
□ GOOD		
□ NEUTRAL	WHAT TIME DID YOU GO TO BED?	
□ STRESSED	□ AM □ PM	

SELF CARE TRACKER

MIND / SPIRIT	EXERCISE / PHYSICAL ACTIVITY

MINDFULNESS

POSITIVE AFFIRMATIONS	GRATITUDE

MEDITATION LOG

DATE		TIME		HOW LONG	

MOOD TRACKER

BEFORE	AFTER	THOUGHTS / NOTES ON YOUR MEDITATION
□ GOOD	□ GOOD	
□ NEUTRAL	□ NEUTRAL	
□ STRESSED	□ STRESSED	

SLEEP TRACKER

SLEEP QUALITY	HOW MANY HOURS DID YOU SLEEP?	DREAM NOTES
□ GOOD		
□ NEUTRAL	WHAT TIME DID YOU GO TO BED?	
□ STRESSED	□ AM □ PM	

SELF CARE TRACKER

MIND / SPIRIT	EXERCISE / PHYSICAL ACTIVITY

MINDFULNESS

POSITIVE AFFIRMATIONS	GRATITUDE

MEDITATION LOG

DATE		TIME		HOW LONG	

MOOD TRACKER

BEFORE	AFTER	THOUGHTS / NOTES ON YOUR MEDITATION
□ GOOD	□ GOOD	
□ NEUTRAL	□ NEUTRAL	
□ STRESSED	□ STRESSED	

SLEEP TRACKER

SLEEP QUALITY	HOW MANY HOURS DID YOU SLEEP?	DREAM NOTES
□ GOOD		
□ NEUTRAL	**WHAT TIME DID YOU GO TO BED?**	
□ STRESSED	□ AM □ PM	

SELF CARE TRACKER

MIND / SPIRIT	EXERCISE / PHYSICAL ACTIVITY

MINDFULNESS

POSITIVE AFFIRMATIONS	GRATITUDE

MEDITATION LOG

DATE		TIME		HOW LONG	

MOOD TRACKER

BEFORE	AFTER	THOUGHTS / NOTES ON YOUR MEDITATION
□ GOOD	□ GOOD	
□ NEUTRAL	□ NEUTRAL	
□ STRESSED	□ STRESSED	

SLEEP TRACKER

SLEEP QUALITY	HOW MANY HOURS DID YOU SLEEP?	DREAM NOTES
□ GOOD		
□ NEUTRAL	**WHAT TIME DID YOU GO TO BED?**	
□ STRESSED	□ AM □ PM	

SELF CARE TRACKER

MIND / SPIRIT	EXERCISE / PHYSICAL ACTIVITY

MINDFULNESS

POSITIVE AFFIRMATIONS	GRATITUDE

MEDITATION LOG

DATE		TIME		HOW LONG	

MOOD TRACKER

BEFORE	AFTER	THOUGHTS / NOTES ON YOUR MEDITATION
□ GOOD	□ GOOD	
□ NEUTRAL	□ NEUTRAL	
□ STRESSED	□ STRESSED	

SLEEP TRACKER

SLEEP QUALITY	HOW MANY HOURS DID YOU SLEEP?	DREAM NOTES
□ GOOD		
□ NEUTRAL	**WHAT TIME DID YOU GO TO BED?**	
□ STRESSED	□ AM □ PM	

SELF CARE TRACKER

MIND / SPIRIT	EXERCISE / PHYSICAL ACTIVITY

MINDFULNESS

POSITIVE AFFIRMATIONS	GRATITUDE

MEDITATION LOG

DATE		TIME		HOW LONG	

MOOD TRACKER

BEFORE	AFTER	THOUGHTS / NOTES ON YOUR MEDITATION
□ GOOD	□ GOOD	
□ NEUTRAL	□ NEUTRAL	
□ STRESSED	□ STRESSED	

SLEEP TRACKER

SLEEP QUALITY	HOW MANY HOURS DID YOU SLEEP?	DREAM NOTES
□ GOOD		
□ NEUTRAL	WHAT TIME DID YOU GO TO BED?	
□ STRESSED	□ AM □ PM	

SELF CARE TRACKER

MIND / SPIRIT	EXERCISE / PHYSICAL ACTIVITY

MINDFULNESS

POSITIVE AFFIRMATIONS	GRATITUDE

MEDITATION LOG

DATE		TIME		HOW LONG	

MOOD TRACKER

BEFORE	AFTER	THOUGHTS / NOTES ON YOUR MEDITATION
□ GOOD	□ GOOD	
□ NEUTRAL	□ NEUTRAL	
□ STRESSED	□ STRESSED	

SLEEP TRACKER

SLEEP QUALITY	HOW MANY HOURS DID YOU SLEEP?	DREAM NOTES
□ GOOD		
□ NEUTRAL	**WHAT TIME DID YOU GO TO BED?**	
□ STRESSED	□ AM □ PM	

SELF CARE TRACKER

MIND / SPIRIT	EXERCISE / PHYSICAL ACTIVITY

MINDFULNESS

POSITIVE AFFIRMATIONS	GRATITUDE

MEDITATION LOG

DATE		TIME		HOW LONG	

MOOD TRACKER

BEFORE	AFTER	THOUGHTS / NOTES ON YOUR MEDITATION
□ GOOD	□ GOOD	
□ NEUTRAL	□ NEUTRAL	
□ STRESSED	□ STRESSED	

SLEEP TRACKER

SLEEP QUALITY	HOW MANY HOURS DID YOU SLEEP?	DREAM NOTES
□ GOOD		
□ NEUTRAL	WHAT TIME DID YOU GO TO BED?	
□ STRESSED	□ AM □ PM	

SELF CARE TRACKER

MIND / SPIRIT	EXERCISE / PHYSICAL ACTIVITY

MINDFULNESS

POSITIVE AFFIRMATIONS	GRATITUDE

MEDITATION LOG

DATE		TIME		HOW LONG	

MOOD TRACKER

BEFORE	AFTER	THOUGHTS / NOTES ON YOUR MEDITATION
□ GOOD	□ GOOD	
□ NEUTRAL	□ NEUTRAL	
□ STRESSED	□ STRESSED	

SLEEP TRACKER

SLEEP QUALITY	HOW MANY HOURS DID YOU SLEEP?	DREAM NOTES
□ GOOD		
□ NEUTRAL	WHAT TIME DID YOU GO TO BED?	
□ STRESSED	□ AM □ PM	

SELF CARE TRACKER

MIND / SPIRIT	EXERCISE / PHYSICAL ACTIVITY

MINDFULNESS

POSITIVE AFFIRMATIONS	GRATITUDE

MEDITATION LOG

DATE		TIME		HOW LONG	

MOOD TRACKER

BEFORE	AFTER	THOUGHTS / NOTES ON YOUR MEDITATION
□ GOOD	□ GOOD	
□ NEUTRAL	□ NEUTRAL	
□ STRESSED	□ STRESSED	

SLEEP TRACKER

SLEEP QUALITY	HOW MANY HOURS DID YOU SLEEP?	DREAM NOTES
□ GOOD		
□ NEUTRAL	WHAT TIME DID YOU GO TO BED?	
□ STRESSED	□ AM □ PM	

SELF CARE TRACKER

MIND / SPIRIT	EXERCISE / PHYSICAL ACTIVITY

MINDFULNESS

POSITIVE AFFIRMATIONS	GRATITUDE

MEDITATION LOG

DATE		TIME		HOW LONG	

MOOD TRACKER

BEFORE	AFTER	THOUGHTS / NOTES ON YOUR MEDITATION
□ GOOD	□ GOOD	
□ NEUTRAL	□ NEUTRAL	
□ STRESSED	□ STRESSED	

SLEEP TRACKER

SLEEP QUALITY	HOW MANY HOURS DID YOU SLEEP?	DREAM NOTES
□ GOOD		
□ NEUTRAL	**WHAT TIME DID YOU GO TO BED?**	
□ STRESSED	□ AM □ PM	

SELF CARE TRACKER

MIND / SPIRIT	EXERCISE / PHYSICAL ACTIVITY

MINDFULNESS

POSITIVE AFFIRMATIONS	GRATITUDE

MEDITATION LOG

DATE		TIME		HOW LONG	

MOOD TRACKER

BEFORE	AFTER	THOUGHTS / NOTES ON YOUR MEDITATION
□ GOOD	□ GOOD	
□ NEUTRAL	□ NEUTRAL	
□ STRESSED	□ STRESSED	

SLEEP TRACKER

SLEEP QUALITY	HOW MANY HOURS DID YOU SLEEP?	DREAM NOTES
□ GOOD		
□ NEUTRAL	WHAT TIME DID YOU GO TO BED?	
□ STRESSED	□ AM □ PM	

SELF CARE TRACKER

MIND / SPIRIT	EXERCISE / PHYSICAL ACTIVITY

MINDFULNESS

POSITIVE AFFIRMATIONS	GRATITUDE

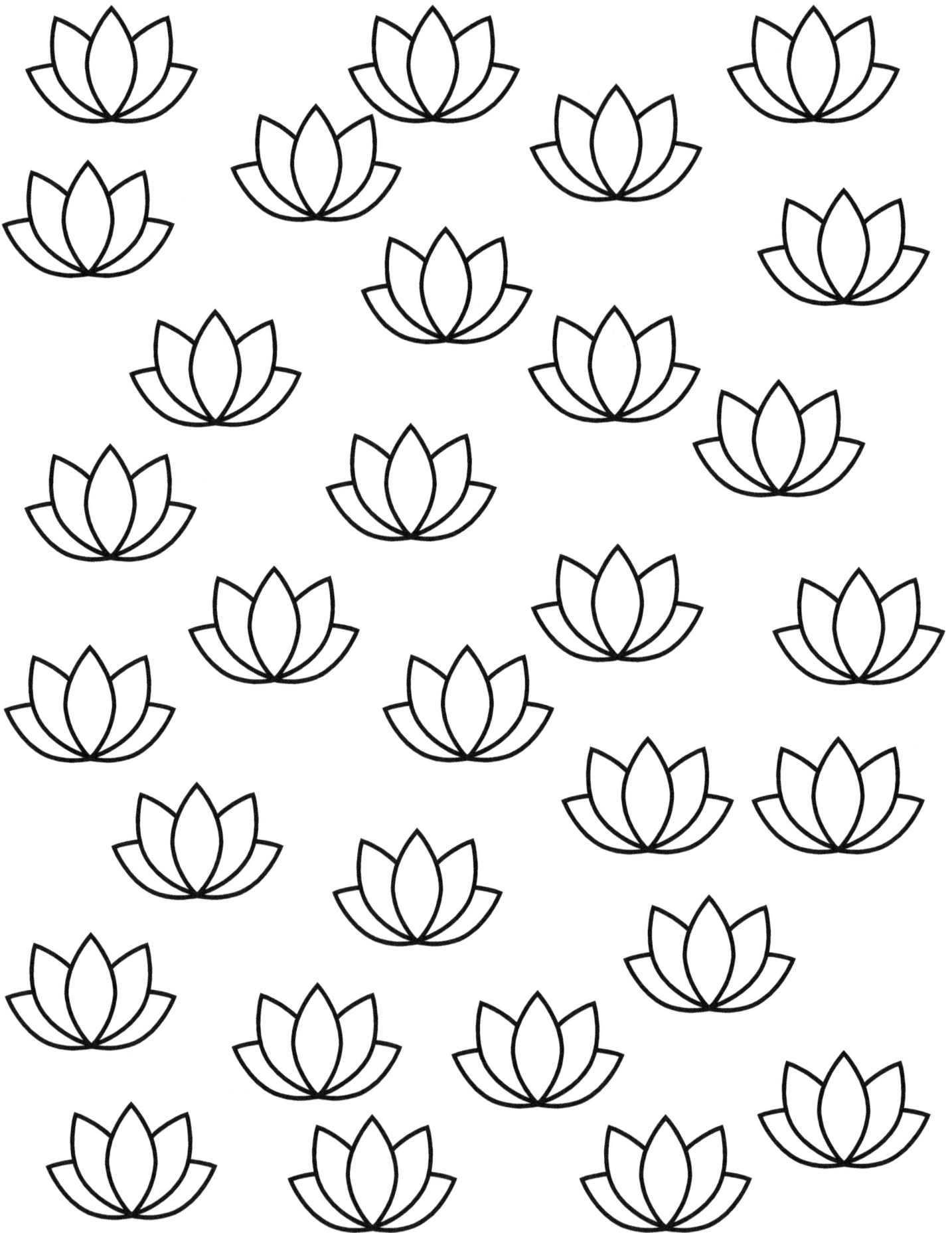

MEDITATION LOG

DATE		TIME		HOW LONG	

MOOD TRACKER

BEFORE	AFTER	THOUGHTS / NOTES ON YOUR MEDITATION
□ GOOD	□ GOOD	
□ NEUTRAL	□ NEUTRAL	
□ STRESSED	□ STRESSED	

SLEEP TRACKER

SLEEP QUALITY	HOW MANY HOURS DID YOU SLEEP?	DREAM NOTES
□ GOOD		
□ NEUTRAL	WHAT TIME DID YOU GO TO BED?	
□ STRESSED	□ AM □ PM	

SELF CARE TRACKER

MIND / SPIRIT	EXERCISE / PHYSICAL ACTIVITY

MINDFULNESS

POSITIVE AFFIRMATIONS	GRATITUDE

MEDITATION LOG

DATE		TIME		HOW LONG	

MOOD TRACKER

BEFORE	AFTER	THOUGHTS / NOTES ON YOUR MEDITATION
□ GOOD	□ GOOD	
□ NEUTRAL	□ NEUTRAL	
□ STRESSED	□ STRESSED	

SLEEP TRACKER

SLEEP QUALITY	HOW MANY HOURS DID YOU SLEEP?	DREAM NOTES
□ GOOD		
□ NEUTRAL	WHAT TIME DID YOU GO TO BED?	
□ STRESSED	□ AM □ PM	

SELF CARE TRACKER

MIND / SPIRIT	EXERCISE / PHYSICAL ACTIVITY

MINDFULNESS

POSITIVE AFFIRMATIONS	GRATITUDE

MEDITATION LOG

DATE		TIME		HOW LONG	

MOOD TRACKER

BEFORE	AFTER	THOUGHTS / NOTES ON YOUR MEDITATION
□ GOOD	□ GOOD	
□ NEUTRAL	□ NEUTRAL	
□ STRESSED	□ STRESSED	

SLEEP TRACKER

SLEEP QUALITY	HOW MANY HOURS DID YOU SLEEP?	DREAM NOTES
□ GOOD		
□ NEUTRAL	WHAT TIME DID YOU GO TO BED?	
□ STRESSED	□ AM □ PM	

SELF CARE TRACKER

MIND / SPIRIT	EXERCISE / PHYSICAL ACTIVITY

MINDFULNESS

POSITIVE AFFIRMATIONS	GRATITUDE

MEDITATION LOG

DATE		TIME		HOW LONG	

MOOD TRACKER

BEFORE	AFTER	THOUGHTS / NOTES ON YOUR MEDITATION
□ GOOD	□ GOOD	
□ NEUTRAL	□ NEUTRAL	
□ STRESSED	□ STRESSED	

SLEEP TRACKER

SLEEP QUALITY	HOW MANY HOURS DID YOU SLEEP?	DREAM NOTES
□ GOOD		
□ NEUTRAL	WHAT TIME DID YOU GO TO BED?	
□ STRESSED	□ AM □ PM	

SELF CARE TRACKER

MIND / SPIRIT	EXERCISE / PHYSICAL ACTIVITY

MINDFULNESS

POSITIVE AFFIRMATIONS	GRATITUDE

MEDITATION LOG

DATE		TIME		HOW LONG	

MOOD TRACKER

BEFORE	AFTER	THOUGHTS / NOTES ON YOUR MEDITATION
□ GOOD	□ GOOD	
□ NEUTRAL	□ NEUTRAL	
□ STRESSED	□ STRESSED	

SLEEP TRACKER

SLEEP QUALITY	HOW MANY HOURS DID YOU SLEEP?	DREAM NOTES
□ GOOD		
□ NEUTRAL	WHAT TIME DID YOU GO TO BED?	
□ STRESSED	□ AM □ PM	

SELF CARE TRACKER

MIND / SPIRIT	EXERCISE / PHYSICAL ACTIVITY

MINDFULNESS

POSITIVE AFFIRMATIONS	GRATITUDE

MEDITATION LOG

DATE		TIME		HOW LONG	

MOOD TRACKER

BEFORE	AFTER	THOUGHTS / NOTES ON YOUR MEDITATION
□ GOOD	□ GOOD	
□ NEUTRAL	□ NEUTRAL	
□ STRESSED	□ STRESSED	

SLEEP TRACKER

SLEEP QUALITY	HOW MANY HOURS DID YOU SLEEP?	DREAM NOTES
□ GOOD		
□ NEUTRAL	WHAT TIME DID YOU GO TO BED?	
□ STRESSED	□ AM □ PM	

SELF CARE TRACKER

MIND / SPIRIT	EXERCISE / PHYSICAL ACTIVITY

MINDFULNESS

POSITIVE AFFIRMATIONS	GRATITUDE

MEDITATION LOG

DATE		TIME		HOW LONG	

MOOD TRACKER

BEFORE	AFTER	THOUGHTS / NOTES ON YOUR MEDITATION
□ GOOD	□ GOOD	
□ NEUTRAL	□ NEUTRAL	
□ STRESSED	□ STRESSED	

SLEEP TRACKER

SLEEP QUALITY	HOW MANY HOURS DID YOU SLEEP?	DREAM NOTES
□ GOOD		
□ NEUTRAL	**WHAT TIME DID YOU GO TO BED?**	
□ STRESSED	□ AM □ PM	

SELF CARE TRACKER

MIND / SPIRIT	EXERCISE / PHYSICAL ACTIVITY

MINDFULNESS

POSITIVE AFFIRMATIONS	GRATITUDE

MEDITATION LOG

DATE		TIME		HOW LONG	

MOOD TRACKER

BEFORE	AFTER	THOUGHTS / NOTES ON YOUR MEDITATION
□ GOOD	□ GOOD	
□ NEUTRAL	□ NEUTRAL	
□ STRESSED	□ STRESSED	

SLEEP TRACKER

SLEEP QUALITY	HOW MANY HOURS DID YOU SLEEP?	DREAM NOTES
□ GOOD		
□ NEUTRAL	WHAT TIME DID YOU GO TO BED?	
□ STRESSED	□ AM □ PM	

SELF CARE TRACKER

MIND / SPIRIT	EXERCISE / PHYSICAL ACTIVITY

MINDFULNESS

POSITIVE AFFIRMATIONS	GRATITUDE

MEDITATION LOG

DATE		TIME		HOW LONG	

MOOD TRACKER

BEFORE	AFTER	THOUGHTS / NOTES ON YOUR MEDITATION
□ GOOD	□ GOOD	
□ NEUTRAL	□ NEUTRAL	
□ STRESSED	□ STRESSED	

SLEEP TRACKER

SLEEP QUALITY	HOW MANY HOURS DID YOU SLEEP?	DREAM NOTES
□ GOOD		
□ NEUTRAL	WHAT TIME DID YOU GO TO BED?	
□ STRESSED	□ AM □ PM	

SELF CARE TRACKER

MIND / SPIRIT	EXERCISE / PHYSICAL ACTIVITY

MINDFULNESS

POSITIVE AFFIRMATIONS	GRATITUDE

MEDITATION LOG

DATE		TIME		HOW LONG	

MOOD TRACKER

BEFORE	AFTER	THOUGHTS / NOTES ON YOUR MEDITATION
□ GOOD	□ GOOD	
□ NEUTRAL	□ NEUTRAL	
□ STRESSED	□ STRESSED	

SLEEP TRACKER

SLEEP QUALITY	HOW MANY HOURS DID YOU SLEEP?	DREAM NOTES
□ GOOD		
□ NEUTRAL	WHAT TIME DID YOU GO TO BED?	
□ STRESSED	□ AM □ PM	

SELF CARE TRACKER

MIND / SPIRIT	EXERCISE / PHYSICAL ACTIVITY

MINDFULNESS

POSITIVE AFFIRMATIONS	GRATITUDE

MEDITATION LOG

DATE		TIME		HOW LONG	

MOOD TRACKER

BEFORE	AFTER	THOUGHTS / NOTES ON YOUR MEDITATION
□ GOOD	□ GOOD	
□ NEUTRAL	□ NEUTRAL	
□ STRESSED	□ STRESSED	

SLEEP TRACKER

SLEEP QUALITY	HOW MANY HOURS DID YOU SLEEP?	DREAM NOTES
□ GOOD		
□ NEUTRAL	WHAT TIME DID YOU GO TO BED?	
□ STRESSED	□ AM □ PM	

SELF CARE TRACKER

MIND / SPIRIT	EXERCISE / PHYSICAL ACTIVITY

MINDFULNESS

POSITIVE AFFIRMATIONS	GRATITUDE

MEDITATION LOG

DATE		TIME		HOW LONG	

MOOD TRACKER

BEFORE	AFTER	THOUGHTS / NOTES ON YOUR MEDITATION
□ GOOD	□ GOOD	
□ NEUTRAL	□ NEUTRAL	
□ STRESSED	□ STRESSED	

SLEEP TRACKER

SLEEP QUALITY	HOW MANY HOURS DID YOU SLEEP?	DREAM NOTES
□ GOOD		
□ NEUTRAL	WHAT TIME DID YOU GO TO BED?	
□ STRESSED	□ AM □ PM	

SELF CARE TRACKER

MIND / SPIRIT	EXERCISE / PHYSICAL ACTIVITY

MINDFULNESS

POSITIVE AFFIRMATIONS	GRATITUDE

MEDITATION LOG

DATE		TIME		HOW LONG	

MOOD TRACKER

BEFORE	AFTER	THOUGHTS / NOTES ON YOUR MEDITATION
□ GOOD	□ GOOD	
□ NEUTRAL	□ NEUTRAL	
□ STRESSED	□ STRESSED	

SLEEP TRACKER

SLEEP QUALITY	HOW MANY HOURS DID YOU SLEEP?	DREAM NOTES
□ GOOD		
□ NEUTRAL	**WHAT TIME DID YOU GO TO BED?**	
□ STRESSED	□ AM □ PM	

SELF CARE TRACKER

MIND / SPIRIT	EXERCISE / PHYSICAL ACTIVITY

MINDFULNESS

POSITIVE AFFIRMATIONS	GRATITUDE

MEDITATION LOG

DATE		TIME		HOW LONG	

MOOD TRACKER

BEFORE	AFTER	THOUGHTS / NOTES ON YOUR MEDITATION
□ GOOD	□ GOOD	
□ NEUTRAL	□ NEUTRAL	
□ STRESSED	□ STRESSED	

SLEEP TRACKER

SLEEP QUALITY	HOW MANY HOURS DID YOU SLEEP?	DREAM NOTES
□ GOOD		
□ NEUTRAL	WHAT TIME DID YOU GO TO BED?	
□ STRESSED	□ AM □ PM	

SELF CARE TRACKER

MIND / SPIRIT	EXERCISE / PHYSICAL ACTIVITY

MINDFULNESS

POSITIVE AFFIRMATIONS	GRATITUDE

MEDITATION LOG

DATE		TIME		HOW LONG	

MOOD TRACKER

BEFORE	AFTER	THOUGHTS / NOTES ON YOUR MEDITATION
□ GOOD	□ GOOD	
□ NEUTRAL	□ NEUTRAL	
□ STRESSED	□ STRESSED	

SLEEP TRACKER

SLEEP QUALITY	HOW MANY HOURS DID YOU SLEEP?	DREAM NOTES
□ GOOD		
□ NEUTRAL	**WHAT TIME DID YOU GO TO BED?**	
□ STRESSED	□ AM □ PM	

SELF CARE TRACKER

MIND / SPIRIT	EXERCISE / PHYSICAL ACTIVITY

MINDFULNESS

POSITIVE AFFIRMATIONS	GRATITUDE

MEDITATION LOG

DATE		TIME		HOW LONG	

MOOD TRACKER

BEFORE	AFTER	THOUGHTS / NOTES ON YOUR MEDITATION
□ GOOD	□ GOOD	
□ NEUTRAL	□ NEUTRAL	
□ STRESSED	□ STRESSED	

SLEEP TRACKER

SLEEP QUALITY	HOW MANY HOURS DID YOU SLEEP?	DREAM NOTES
□ GOOD		
□ NEUTRAL	**WHAT TIME DID YOU GO TO BED?**	
□ STRESSED	□ AM □ PM	

SELF CARE TRACKER

MIND / SPIRIT	EXERCISE / PHYSICAL ACTIVITY

MINDFULNESS

POSITIVE AFFIRMATIONS	GRATITUDE

MEDITATION LOG

DATE		TIME		HOW LONG	

MOOD TRACKER

BEFORE	AFTER	THOUGHTS / NOTES ON YOUR MEDITATION
□ GOOD	□ GOOD	
□ NEUTRAL	□ NEUTRAL	
□ STRESSED	□ STRESSED	

SLEEP TRACKER

SLEEP QUALITY	HOW MANY HOURS DID YOU SLEEP?	DREAM NOTES
□ GOOD		
□ NEUTRAL	WHAT TIME DID YOU GO TO BED?	
□ STRESSED	□ AM □ PM	

SELF CARE TRACKER

MIND / SPIRIT	EXERCISE / PHYSICAL ACTIVITY

MINDFULNESS

POSITIVE AFFIRMATIONS	GRATITUDE

MEDITATION LOG

DATE		TIME		HOW LONG	

MOOD TRACKER

BEFORE	AFTER	THOUGHTS / NOTES ON YOUR MEDITATION
□ GOOD	□ GOOD	
□ NEUTRAL	□ NEUTRAL	
□ STRESSED	□ STRESSED	

SLEEP TRACKER

SLEEP QUALITY	HOW MANY HOURS DID YOU SLEEP?	DREAM NOTES
□ GOOD		
□ NEUTRAL	WHAT TIME DID YOU GO TO BED?	
□ STRESSED	□ AM □ PM	

SELF CARE TRACKER

MIND / SPIRIT	EXERCISE / PHYSICAL ACTIVITY

MINDFULNESS

POSITIVE AFFIRMATIONS	GRATITUDE

MEDITATION LOG

DATE		TIME		HOW LONG	

MOOD TRACKER

BEFORE	AFTER	THOUGHTS / NOTES ON YOUR MEDITATION
□ GOOD	□ GOOD	
□ NEUTRAL	□ NEUTRAL	
□ STRESSED	□ STRESSED	

SLEEP TRACKER

SLEEP QUALITY	HOW MANY HOURS DID YOU SLEEP?	DREAM NOTES
□ GOOD		
□ NEUTRAL	**WHAT TIME DID YOU GO TO BED?**	
□ STRESSED	□ AM □ PM	

SELF CARE TRACKER

MIND / SPIRIT	EXERCISE / PHYSICAL ACTIVITY

MINDFULNESS

POSITIVE AFFIRMATIONS	GRATITUDE

MEDITATION LOG

DATE		TIME		HOW LONG	

MOOD TRACKER

BEFORE	AFTER	THOUGHTS / NOTES ON YOUR MEDITATION
□ GOOD	□ GOOD	
□ NEUTRAL	□ NEUTRAL	
□ STRESSED	□ STRESSED	

SLEEP TRACKER

SLEEP QUALITY	HOW MANY HOURS DID YOU SLEEP?	DREAM NOTES
□ GOOD		
□ NEUTRAL	**WHAT TIME DID YOU GO TO BED?**	
□ STRESSED	□ AM □ PM	

SELF CARE TRACKER

MIND / SPIRIT	EXERCISE / PHYSICAL ACTIVITY

MINDFULNESS

POSITIVE AFFIRMATIONS	GRATITUDE

MEDITATION LOG

DATE		TIME		HOW LONG	

MOOD TRACKER

BEFORE	AFTER	THOUGHTS / NOTES ON YOUR MEDITATION
□ GOOD	□ GOOD	
□ NEUTRAL	□ NEUTRAL	
□ STRESSED	□ STRESSED	

SLEEP TRACKER

SLEEP QUALITY	HOW MANY HOURS DID YOU SLEEP?	DREAM NOTES
□ GOOD		
□ NEUTRAL	**WHAT TIME DID YOU GO TO BED?**	
□ STRESSED	□ AM □ PM	

SELF CARE TRACKER

MIND / SPIRIT	EXERCISE / PHYSICAL ACTIVITY

MINDFULNESS

POSITIVE AFFIRMATIONS	GRATITUDE

MEDITATION LOG

DATE		TIME		HOW LONG	

MOOD TRACKER

BEFORE	AFTER	THOUGHTS / NOTES ON YOUR MEDITATION
□ GOOD	□ GOOD	
□ NEUTRAL	□ NEUTRAL	
□ STRESSED	□ STRESSED	

SLEEP TRACKER

SLEEP QUALITY	HOW MANY HOURS DID YOU SLEEP?	DREAM NOTES
□ GOOD		
□ NEUTRAL	WHAT TIME DID YOU GO TO BED?	
□ STRESSED	□ AM □ PM	

SELF CARE TRACKER

MIND / SPIRIT	EXERCISE / PHYSICAL ACTIVITY

MINDFULNESS

POSITIVE AFFIRMATIONS	GRATITUDE

MEDITATION LOG

DATE		TIME		HOW LONG	

MOOD TRACKER

BEFORE	AFTER	THOUGHTS / NOTES ON YOUR MEDITATION
□ GOOD	□ GOOD	
□ NEUTRAL	□ NEUTRAL	
□ STRESSED	□ STRESSED	

SLEEP TRACKER

SLEEP QUALITY	HOW MANY HOURS DID YOU SLEEP?	DREAM NOTES
□ GOOD		
□ NEUTRAL	**WHAT TIME DID YOU GO TO BED?**	
□ STRESSED	□ AM □ PM	

SELF CARE TRACKER

MIND / SPIRIT	EXERCISE / PHYSICAL ACTIVITY

MINDFULNESS

POSITIVE AFFIRMATIONS	GRATITUDE

MEDITATION LOG

DATE		TIME		HOW LONG	

MOOD TRACKER

BEFORE	AFTER	THOUGHTS / NOTES ON YOUR MEDITATION
□ GOOD	□ GOOD	
□ NEUTRAL	□ NEUTRAL	
□ STRESSED	□ STRESSED	

SLEEP TRACKER

SLEEP QUALITY	HOW MANY HOURS DID YOU SLEEP?	DREAM NOTES
□ GOOD		
□ NEUTRAL	WHAT TIME DID YOU GO TO BED?	
□ STRESSED	□ AM □ PM	

SELF CARE TRACKER

MIND / SPIRIT	EXERCISE / PHYSICAL ACTIVITY

MINDFULNESS

POSITIVE AFFIRMATIONS	GRATITUDE

MEDITATION LOG

DATE		TIME		HOW LONG	

MOOD TRACKER

BEFORE	AFTER	THOUGHTS / NOTES ON YOUR MEDITATION
□ GOOD	□ GOOD	
□ NEUTRAL	□ NEUTRAL	
□ STRESSED	□ STRESSED	

SLEEP TRACKER

SLEEP QUALITY	HOW MANY HOURS DID YOU SLEEP?	DREAM NOTES
□ GOOD		
□ NEUTRAL	WHAT TIME DID YOU GO TO BED?	
□ STRESSED	□ AM □ PM	

SELF CARE TRACKER

MIND / SPIRIT	EXERCISE / PHYSICAL ACTIVITY

MINDFULNESS

POSITIVE AFFIRMATIONS	GRATITUDE

MEDITATION LOG

DATE		TIME		HOW LONG	

MOOD TRACKER

BEFORE	AFTER	THOUGHTS / NOTES ON YOUR MEDITATION
□ GOOD	□ GOOD	
□ NEUTRAL	□ NEUTRAL	
□ STRESSED	□ STRESSED	

SLEEP TRACKER

SLEEP QUALITY	HOW MANY HOURS DID YOU SLEEP?	DREAM NOTES
□ GOOD		
□ NEUTRAL	WHAT TIME DID YOU GO TO BED?	
□ STRESSED	□ AM □ PM	

SELF CARE TRACKER

MIND / SPIRIT	EXERCISE / PHYSICAL ACTIVITY

MINDFULNESS

POSITIVE AFFIRMATIONS	GRATITUDE

MEDITATION LOG

DATE		TIME		HOW LONG	

MOOD TRACKER

BEFORE	AFTER	THOUGHTS / NOTES ON YOUR MEDITATION
□ GOOD	□ GOOD	
□ NEUTRAL	□ NEUTRAL	
□ STRESSED	□ STRESSED	

SLEEP TRACKER

SLEEP QUALITY	HOW MANY HOURS DID YOU SLEEP?	DREAM NOTES
□ GOOD		
□ NEUTRAL	WHAT TIME DID YOU GO TO BED?	
□ STRESSED	□ AM □ PM	

SELF CARE TRACKER

MIND / SPIRIT	EXERCISE / PHYSICAL ACTIVITY

MINDFULNESS

POSITIVE AFFIRMATIONS	GRATITUDE

MEDITATION LOG

DATE		TIME		HOW LONG	

MOOD TRACKER

BEFORE	AFTER	THOUGHTS / NOTES ON YOUR MEDITATION
□ GOOD	□ GOOD	
□ NEUTRAL	□ NEUTRAL	
□ STRESSED	□ STRESSED	

SLEEP TRACKER

SLEEP QUALITY	HOW MANY HOURS DID YOU SLEEP?	DREAM NOTES
□ GOOD		
□ NEUTRAL	WHAT TIME DID YOU GO TO BED?	
□ STRESSED	□ AM □ PM	

SELF CARE TRACKER

MIND / SPIRIT	EXERCISE / PHYSICAL ACTIVITY

MINDFULNESS

POSITIVE AFFIRMATIONS	GRATITUDE

MEDITATION LOG

DATE		TIME		HOW LONG	

MOOD TRACKER

BEFORE	AFTER	THOUGHTS / NOTES ON YOUR MEDITATION
□ GOOD	□ GOOD	
□ NEUTRAL	□ NEUTRAL	
□ STRESSED	□ STRESSED	

SLEEP TRACKER

SLEEP QUALITY	HOW MANY HOURS DID YOU SLEEP?	DREAM NOTES
□ GOOD		
□ NEUTRAL	WHAT TIME DID YOU GO TO BED?	
□ STRESSED	□ AM □ PM	

SELF CARE TRACKER

MIND / SPIRIT	EXERCISE / PHYSICAL ACTIVITY

MINDFULNESS

POSITIVE AFFIRMATIONS	GRATITUDE

MEDITATION LOG

DATE		TIME		HOW LONG	

MOOD TRACKER

BEFORE	AFTER	THOUGHTS / NOTES ON YOUR MEDITATION
□ GOOD	□ GOOD	
□ NEUTRAL	□ NEUTRAL	
□ STRESSED	□ STRESSED	

SLEEP TRACKER

SLEEP QUALITY	HOW MANY HOURS DID YOU SLEEP?	DREAM NOTES
□ GOOD		
□ NEUTRAL	WHAT TIME DID YOU GO TO BED?	
□ STRESSED	□ AM □ PM	

SELF CARE TRACKER

MIND / SPIRIT	EXERCISE / PHYSICAL ACTIVITY

MINDFULNESS

POSITIVE AFFIRMATIONS	GRATITUDE

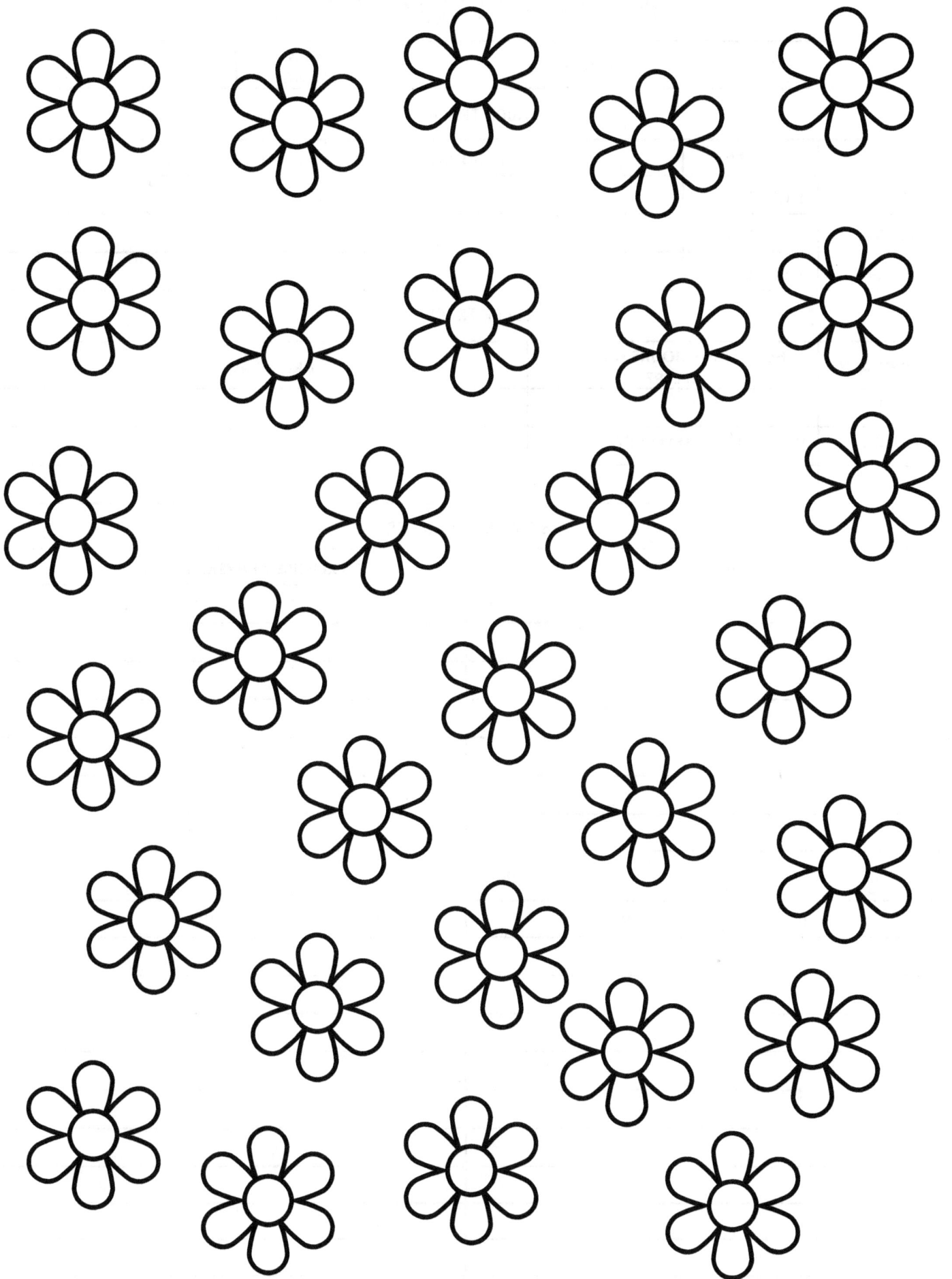

MEDITATION LOG

DATE		TIME		HOW LONG	

MOOD TRACKER

BEFORE	AFTER	THOUGHTS / NOTES ON YOUR MEDITATION
□ GOOD	□ GOOD	
□ NEUTRAL	□ NEUTRAL	
□ STRESSED	□ STRESSED	

SLEEP TRACKER

SLEEP QUALITY	HOW MANY HOURS DID YOU SLEEP?	DREAM NOTES
□ GOOD		
□ NEUTRAL	WHAT TIME DID YOU GO TO BED?	
□ STRESSED	□ AM □ PM	

SELF CARE TRACKER

MIND / SPIRIT	EXERCISE / PHYSICAL ACTIVITY

MINDFULNESS

POSITIVE AFFIRMATIONS	GRATITUDE

MEDITATION LOG

DATE		TIME		HOW LONG	

MOOD TRACKER

BEFORE	AFTER	THOUGHTS / NOTES ON YOUR MEDITATION
□ GOOD	□ GOOD	
□ NEUTRAL	□ NEUTRAL	
□ STRESSED	□ STRESSED	

SLEEP TRACKER

SLEEP QUALITY	HOW MANY HOURS DID YOU SLEEP?	DREAM NOTES
□ GOOD		
□ NEUTRAL	WHAT TIME DID YOU GO TO BED?	
□ STRESSED	□ AM □ PM	

SELF CARE TRACKER

MIND / SPIRIT	EXERCISE / PHYSICAL ACTIVITY

MINDFULNESS

POSITIVE AFFIRMATIONS	GRATITUDE

MEDITATION LOG

DATE		TIME		HOW LONG	

MOOD TRACKER

BEFORE	AFTER	THOUGHTS / NOTES ON YOUR MEDITATION
□ GOOD	□ GOOD	
□ NEUTRAL	□ NEUTRAL	
□ STRESSED	□ STRESSED	

SLEEP TRACKER

SLEEP QUALITY	HOW MANY HOURS DID YOU SLEEP?	DREAM NOTES
□ GOOD		
□ NEUTRAL	WHAT TIME DID YOU GO TO BED?	
□ STRESSED	□ AM □ PM	

SELF CARE TRACKER

MIND / SPIRIT	EXERCISE / PHYSICAL ACTIVITY

MINDFULNESS

POSITIVE AFFIRMATIONS	GRATITUDE

MEDITATION LOG

DATE		TIME		HOW LONG	

MOOD TRACKER

BEFORE	AFTER	THOUGHTS / NOTES ON YOUR MEDITATION
□ GOOD	□ GOOD	
□ NEUTRAL	□ NEUTRAL	
□ STRESSED	□ STRESSED	

SLEEP TRACKER

SLEEP QUALITY	HOW MANY HOURS DID YOU SLEEP?	DREAM NOTES
□ GOOD		
□ NEUTRAL	**WHAT TIME DID YOU GO TO BED?**	
□ STRESSED	□ AM □ PM	

SELF CARE TRACKER

MIND / SPIRIT	EXERCISE / PHYSICAL ACTIVITY

MINDFULNESS

POSITIVE AFFIRMATIONS	GRATITUDE

MEDITATION LOG

DATE		TIME		HOW LONG	

MOOD TRACKER

BEFORE	AFTER	THOUGHTS / NOTES ON YOUR MEDITATION
□ GOOD	□ GOOD	
□ NEUTRAL	□ NEUTRAL	
□ STRESSED	□ STRESSED	

SLEEP TRACKER

SLEEP QUALITY	HOW MANY HOURS DID YOU SLEEP?	DREAM NOTES
□ GOOD		
□ NEUTRAL	WHAT TIME DID YOU GO TO BED?	
□ STRESSED	□ AM □ PM	

SELF CARE TRACKER

MIND / SPIRIT	EXERCISE / PHYSICAL ACTIVITY

MINDFULNESS

POSITIVE AFFIRMATIONS	GRATITUDE

MEDITATION LOG

DATE		TIME		HOW LONG	

MOOD TRACKER

BEFORE	AFTER	THOUGHTS / NOTES ON YOUR MEDITATION
□ GOOD	□ GOOD	
□ NEUTRAL	□ NEUTRAL	
□ STRESSED	□ STRESSED	

SLEEP TRACKER

SLEEP QUALITY	HOW MANY HOURS DID YOU SLEEP?	DREAM NOTES
□ GOOD		
□ NEUTRAL	WHAT TIME DID YOU GO TO BED?	
□ STRESSED	□ AM □ PM	

SELF CARE TRACKER

MIND / SPIRIT	EXERCISE / PHYSICAL ACTIVITY

MINDFULNESS

POSITIVE AFFIRMATIONS	GRATITUDE

MEDITATION LOG

DATE		TIME		HOW LONG	

MOOD TRACKER

BEFORE	AFTER	THOUGHTS / NOTES ON YOUR MEDITATION
□ GOOD	□ GOOD	
□ NEUTRAL	□ NEUTRAL	
□ STRESSED	□ STRESSED	

SLEEP TRACKER

SLEEP QUALITY	HOW MANY HOURS DID YOU SLEEP?	DREAM NOTES
□ GOOD		
□ NEUTRAL	WHAT TIME DID YOU GO TO BED?	
□ STRESSED	□ AM □ PM	

SELF CARE TRACKER

MIND / SPIRIT	EXERCISE / PHYSICAL ACTIVITY

MINDFULNESS

POSITIVE AFFIRMATIONS	GRATITUDE

MEDITATION LOG

DATE		TIME		HOW LONG	

MOOD TRACKER

BEFORE	AFTER	THOUGHTS / NOTES ON YOUR MEDITATION
□ GOOD	□ GOOD	
□ NEUTRAL	□ NEUTRAL	
□ STRESSED	□ STRESSED	

SLEEP TRACKER

SLEEP QUALITY	HOW MANY HOURS DID YOU SLEEP?	DREAM NOTES
□ GOOD		
□ NEUTRAL	WHAT TIME DID YOU GO TO BED?	
□ STRESSED	□ AM □ PM	

SELF CARE TRACKER

MIND / SPIRIT	EXERCISE / PHYSICAL ACTIVITY

MINDFULNESS

POSITIVE AFFIRMATIONS	GRATITUDE

MEDITATION LOG

DATE		TIME		HOW LONG	

MOOD TRACKER

BEFORE	AFTER	THOUGHTS / NOTES ON YOUR MEDITATION
□ GOOD	□ GOOD	
□ NEUTRAL	□ NEUTRAL	
□ STRESSED	□ STRESSED	

SLEEP TRACKER

SLEEP QUALITY	HOW MANY HOURS DID YOU SLEEP?	DREAM NOTES
□ GOOD		
□ NEUTRAL	WHAT TIME DID YOU GO TO BED?	
□ STRESSED	□ AM □ PM	

SELF CARE TRACKER

MIND / SPIRIT	EXERCISE / PHYSICAL ACTIVITY

MINDFULNESS

POSITIVE AFFIRMATIONS	GRATITUDE

MEDITATION LOG

DATE		TIME		HOW LONG	

MOOD TRACKER

BEFORE	AFTER	THOUGHTS / NOTES ON YOUR MEDITATION
□ GOOD	□ GOOD	
□ NEUTRAL	□ NEUTRAL	
□ STRESSED	□ STRESSED	

SLEEP TRACKER

SLEEP QUALITY	HOW MANY HOURS DID YOU SLEEP?	DREAM NOTES
□ GOOD		
□ NEUTRAL	**WHAT TIME DID YOU GO TO BED?**	
□ STRESSED	□ AM □ PM	

SELF CARE TRACKER

MIND / SPIRIT	EXERCISE / PHYSICAL ACTIVITY

MINDFULNESS

POSITIVE AFFIRMATIONS	GRATITUDE

MEDITATION LOG

DATE		TIME		HOW LONG	

MOOD TRACKER

BEFORE	AFTER	THOUGHTS / NOTES ON YOUR MEDITATION
□ GOOD	□ GOOD	
□ NEUTRAL	□ NEUTRAL	
□ STRESSED	□ STRESSED	

SLEEP TRACKER

SLEEP QUALITY	HOW MANY HOURS DID YOU SLEEP?	DREAM NOTES
□ GOOD		
□ NEUTRAL	WHAT TIME DID YOU GO TO BED?	
□ STRESSED	□ AM □ PM	

SELF CARE TRACKER

MIND / SPIRIT	EXERCISE / PHYSICAL ACTIVITY

MINDFULNESS

POSITIVE AFFIRMATIONS	GRATITUDE

MEDITATION LOG

DATE		TIME		HOW LONG	

MOOD TRACKER

BEFORE	AFTER	THOUGHTS / NOTES ON YOUR MEDITATION
□ GOOD	□ GOOD	
□ NEUTRAL	□ NEUTRAL	
□ STRESSED	□ STRESSED	

SLEEP TRACKER

SLEEP QUALITY	HOW MANY HOURS DID YOU SLEEP?	DREAM NOTES
□ GOOD		
□ NEUTRAL	WHAT TIME DID YOU GO TO BED?	
□ STRESSED	□ AM □ PM	

SELF CARE TRACKER

MIND / SPIRIT	EXERCISE / PHYSICAL ACTIVITY

MINDFULNESS

POSITIVE AFFIRMATIONS	GRATITUDE

MEDITATION LOG

DATE		TIME		HOW LONG	

MOOD TRACKER

BEFORE	AFTER	THOUGHTS / NOTES ON YOUR MEDITATION
□ GOOD	□ GOOD	
□ NEUTRAL	□ NEUTRAL	
□ STRESSED	□ STRESSED	

SLEEP TRACKER

SLEEP QUALITY	HOW MANY HOURS DID YOU SLEEP?	DREAM NOTES
□ GOOD		
□ NEUTRAL	WHAT TIME DID YOU GO TO BED?	
□ STRESSED	□ AM □ PM	

SELF CARE TRACKER

MIND / SPIRIT	EXERCISE / PHYSICAL ACTIVITY

MINDFULNESS

POSITIVE AFFIRMATIONS	GRATITUDE

MEDITATION LOG

DATE		TIME		HOW LONG	

MOOD TRACKER

BEFORE	AFTER	THOUGHTS / NOTES ON YOUR MEDITATION
□ GOOD	□ GOOD	
□ NEUTRAL	□ NEUTRAL	
□ STRESSED	□ STRESSED	

SLEEP TRACKER

SLEEP QUALITY	HOW MANY HOURS DID YOU SLEEP?	DREAM NOTES
□ GOOD		
□ NEUTRAL	**WHAT TIME DID YOU GO TO BED?**	
□ STRESSED	□ AM □ PM	

SELF CARE TRACKER

MIND / SPIRIT	EXERCISE / PHYSICAL ACTIVITY

MINDFULNESS

POSITIVE AFFIRMATIONS	GRATITUDE

MEDITATION LOG

DATE		TIME		HOW LONG	

MOOD TRACKER

BEFORE	AFTER	THOUGHTS / NOTES ON YOUR MEDITATION
□ GOOD	□ GOOD	
□ NEUTRAL	□ NEUTRAL	
□ STRESSED	□ STRESSED	

SLEEP TRACKER

SLEEP QUALITY	HOW MANY HOURS DID YOU SLEEP?	DREAM NOTES
□ GOOD		
□ NEUTRAL	WHAT TIME DID YOU GO TO BED?	
□ STRESSED	□ AM □ PM	

SELF CARE TRACKER

MIND / SPIRIT	EXERCISE / PHYSICAL ACTIVITY

MINDFULNESS

POSITIVE AFFIRMATIONS	GRATITUDE

MEDITATION LOG

DATE		TIME		HOW LONG	

MOOD TRACKER

BEFORE	AFTER	THOUGHTS / NOTES ON YOUR MEDITATION
□ GOOD	□ GOOD	
□ NEUTRAL	□ NEUTRAL	
□ STRESSED	□ STRESSED	

SLEEP TRACKER

SLEEP QUALITY	HOW MANY HOURS DID YOU SLEEP?	DREAM NOTES
□ GOOD		
□ NEUTRAL	WHAT TIME DID YOU GO TO BED?	
□ STRESSED	□ AM □ PM	

SELF CARE TRACKER

MIND / SPIRIT	EXERCISE / PHYSICAL ACTIVITY

MINDFULNESS

POSITIVE AFFIRMATIONS	GRATITUDE

MEDITATION LOG

DATE		TIME		HOW LONG	

MOOD TRACKER

BEFORE	AFTER	THOUGHTS / NOTES ON YOUR MEDITATION
□ GOOD	□ GOOD	
□ NEUTRAL	□ NEUTRAL	
□ STRESSED	□ STRESSED	

SLEEP TRACKER

SLEEP QUALITY	HOW MANY HOURS DID YOU SLEEP?	DREAM NOTES
□ GOOD		
□ NEUTRAL	WHAT TIME DID YOU GO TO BED?	
□ STRESSED	□ AM □ PM	

SELF CARE TRACKER

MIND / SPIRIT	EXERCISE / PHYSICAL ACTIVITY

MINDFULNESS

POSITIVE AFFIRMATIONS	GRATITUDE

MEDITATION LOG

DATE		TIME		HOW LONG	

MOOD TRACKER

BEFORE	AFTER	THOUGHTS / NOTES ON YOUR MEDITATION
□ GOOD	□ GOOD	
□ NEUTRAL	□ NEUTRAL	
□ STRESSED	□ STRESSED	

SLEEP TRACKER

SLEEP QUALITY	HOW MANY HOURS DID YOU SLEEP?	DREAM NOTES
□ GOOD		
□ NEUTRAL	WHAT TIME DID YOU GO TO BED?	
□ STRESSED	□ AM □ PM	

SELF CARE TRACKER

MIND / SPIRIT	EXERCISE / PHYSICAL ACTIVITY

MINDFULNESS

POSITIVE AFFIRMATIONS	GRATITUDE

MEDITATION LOG

DATE		TIME		HOW LONG	

MOOD TRACKER

BEFORE	AFTER	THOUGHTS / NOTES ON YOUR MEDITATION
□ GOOD	□ GOOD	
□ NEUTRAL	□ NEUTRAL	
□ STRESSED	□ STRESSED	

SLEEP TRACKER

SLEEP QUALITY	HOW MANY HOURS DID YOU SLEEP?	DREAM NOTES
□ GOOD		
□ NEUTRAL	WHAT TIME DID YOU GO TO BED?	
□ STRESSED	□ AM □ PM	

SELF CARE TRACKER

MIND / SPIRIT	EXERCISE / PHYSICAL ACTIVITY

MINDFULNESS

POSITIVE AFFIRMATIONS	GRATITUDE

MEDITATION LOG

DATE		TIME		HOW LONG	

MOOD TRACKER

BEFORE	AFTER	THOUGHTS / NOTES ON YOUR MEDITATION
□ GOOD	□ GOOD	
□ NEUTRAL	□ NEUTRAL	
□ STRESSED	□ STRESSED	

SLEEP TRACKER

SLEEP QUALITY	HOW MANY HOURS DID YOU SLEEP?	DREAM NOTES
□ GOOD		
□ NEUTRAL	WHAT TIME DID YOU GO TO BED?	
□ STRESSED	□ AM □ PM	

SELF CARE TRACKER

MIND / SPIRIT	EXERCISE / PHYSICAL ACTIVITY

MINDFULNESS

POSITIVE AFFIRMATIONS	GRATITUDE

MEDITATION LOG

DATE		TIME		HOW LONG	

MOOD TRACKER

BEFORE	AFTER	THOUGHTS / NOTES ON YOUR MEDITATION
□ GOOD	□ GOOD	
□ NEUTRAL	□ NEUTRAL	
□ STRESSED	□ STRESSED	

SLEEP TRACKER

SLEEP QUALITY	HOW MANY HOURS DID YOU SLEEP?	DREAM NOTES
□ GOOD		
□ NEUTRAL	**WHAT TIME DID YOU GO TO BED?**	
□ STRESSED	□ AM □ PM	

SELF CARE TRACKER

MIND / SPIRIT	EXERCISE / PHYSICAL ACTIVITY

MINDFULNESS

POSITIVE AFFIRMATIONS	GRATITUDE

MEDITATION LOG

DATE		TIME		HOW LONG	

MOOD TRACKER

BEFORE	AFTER	THOUGHTS / NOTES ON YOUR MEDITATION
□ GOOD	□ GOOD	
□ NEUTRAL	□ NEUTRAL	
□ STRESSED	□ STRESSED	

SLEEP TRACKER

SLEEP QUALITY	HOW MANY HOURS DID YOU SLEEP?	DREAM NOTES
□ GOOD		
□ NEUTRAL	**WHAT TIME DID YOU GO TO BED?**	
□ STRESSED	□ AM □ PM	

SELF CARE TRACKER

MIND / SPIRIT	EXERCISE / PHYSICAL ACTIVITY

MINDFULNESS

POSITIVE AFFIRMATIONS	GRATITUDE

MEDITATION LOG

DATE		TIME		HOW LONG	

MOOD TRACKER

BEFORE	AFTER	THOUGHTS / NOTES ON YOUR MEDITATION
□ GOOD	□ GOOD	
□ NEUTRAL	□ NEUTRAL	
□ STRESSED	□ STRESSED	

SLEEP TRACKER

SLEEP QUALITY	HOW MANY HOURS DID YOU SLEEP?	DREAM NOTES
□ GOOD		
□ NEUTRAL	WHAT TIME DID YOU GO TO BED?	
□ STRESSED	□ AM □ PM	

SELF CARE TRACKER

MIND / SPIRIT	EXERCISE / PHYSICAL ACTIVITY

MINDFULNESS

POSITIVE AFFIRMATIONS	GRATITUDE

MEDITATION LOG

DATE		TIME		HOW LONG	

MOOD TRACKER

BEFORE	AFTER	THOUGHTS / NOTES ON YOUR MEDITATION
□ GOOD	□ GOOD	
□ NEUTRAL	□ NEUTRAL	
□ STRESSED	□ STRESSED	

SLEEP TRACKER

SLEEP QUALITY	HOW MANY HOURS DID YOU SLEEP?	DREAM NOTES
□ GOOD		
□ NEUTRAL	WHAT TIME DID YOU GO TO BED?	
□ STRESSED	□ AM □ PM	

SELF CARE TRACKER

MIND / SPIRIT	EXERCISE / PHYSICAL ACTIVITY

MINDFULNESS

POSITIVE AFFIRMATIONS	GRATITUDE

MEDITATION LOG

DATE		TIME		HOW LONG	

MOOD TRACKER

BEFORE	AFTER	THOUGHTS / NOTES ON YOUR MEDITATION
□ GOOD	□ GOOD	
□ NEUTRAL	□ NEUTRAL	
□ STRESSED	□ STRESSED	

SLEEP TRACKER

SLEEP QUALITY	HOW MANY HOURS DID YOU SLEEP?	DREAM NOTES
□ GOOD		
□ NEUTRAL	WHAT TIME DID YOU GO TO BED?	
□ STRESSED	□ AM □ PM	

SELF CARE TRACKER

MIND / SPIRIT	EXERCISE / PHYSICAL ACTIVITY

MINDFULNESS

POSITIVE AFFIRMATIONS	GRATITUDE

MEDITATION LOG

DATE		TIME		HOW LONG	

MOOD TRACKER

BEFORE	AFTER	THOUGHTS / NOTES ON YOUR MEDITATION
□ GOOD	□ GOOD	
□ NEUTRAL	□ NEUTRAL	
□ STRESSED	□ STRESSED	

SLEEP TRACKER

SLEEP QUALITY	HOW MANY HOURS DID YOU SLEEP?	DREAM NOTES
□ GOOD		
□ NEUTRAL	**WHAT TIME DID YOU GO TO BED?**	
□ STRESSED	□ AM □ PM	

SELF CARE TRACKER

MIND / SPIRIT	EXERCISE / PHYSICAL ACTIVITY

MINDFULNESS

POSITIVE AFFIRMATIONS	GRATITUDE

MEDITATION LOG

DATE		TIME		HOW LONG	

MOOD TRACKER

BEFORE	AFTER	THOUGHTS / NOTES ON YOUR MEDITATION
□ GOOD	□ GOOD	
□ NEUTRAL	□ NEUTRAL	
□ STRESSED	□ STRESSED	

SLEEP TRACKER

SLEEP QUALITY	HOW MANY HOURS DID YOU SLEEP?	DREAM NOTES
□ GOOD		
□ NEUTRAL	WHAT TIME DID YOU GO TO BED?	
□ STRESSED	□ AM □ PM	

SELF CARE TRACKER

MIND / SPIRIT	EXERCISE / PHYSICAL ACTIVITY

MINDFULNESS

POSITIVE AFFIRMATIONS	GRATITUDE

MEDITATION LOG

DATE		TIME		HOW LONG	

MOOD TRACKER

BEFORE	AFTER	THOUGHTS / NOTES ON YOUR MEDITATION
□ GOOD	□ GOOD	
□ NEUTRAL	□ NEUTRAL	
□ STRESSED	□ STRESSED	

SLEEP TRACKER

SLEEP QUALITY	HOW MANY HOURS DID YOU SLEEP?	DREAM NOTES
□ GOOD		
□ NEUTRAL	**WHAT TIME DID YOU GO TO BED?**	
□ STRESSED	□ AM □ PM	

SELF CARE TRACKER

MIND / SPIRIT	EXERCISE / PHYSICAL ACTIVITY

MINDFULNESS

POSITIVE AFFIRMATIONS	GRATITUDE

MEDITATION LOG

DATE		TIME		HOW LONG	

MOOD TRACKER

BEFORE	AFTER	THOUGHTS / NOTES ON YOUR MEDITATION
□ GOOD	□ GOOD	
□ NEUTRAL	□ NEUTRAL	
□ STRESSED	□ STRESSED	

SLEEP TRACKER

SLEEP QUALITY	HOW MANY HOURS DID YOU SLEEP?	DREAM NOTES
□ GOOD		
□ NEUTRAL	WHAT TIME DID YOU GO TO BED?	
□ STRESSED	□ AM □ PM	

SELF CARE TRACKER

MIND / SPIRIT	EXERCISE / PHYSICAL ACTIVITY

MINDFULNESS

POSITIVE AFFIRMATIONS	GRATITUDE

MEDITATION LOG

DATE		TIME		HOW LONG	

MOOD TRACKER

BEFORE	AFTER	THOUGHTS / NOTES ON YOUR MEDITATION
□ GOOD	□ GOOD	
□ NEUTRAL	□ NEUTRAL	
□ STRESSED	□ STRESSED	

SLEEP TRACKER

SLEEP QUALITY	HOW MANY HOURS DID YOU SLEEP?	DREAM NOTES
□ GOOD		
□ NEUTRAL	WHAT TIME DID YOU GO TO BED?	
□ STRESSED	□ AM □ PM	

SELF CARE TRACKER

MIND / SPIRIT	EXERCISE / PHYSICAL ACTIVITY

MINDFULNESS

POSITIVE AFFIRMATIONS	GRATITUDE

MEDITATION LOG

DATE		TIME		HOW LONG	

MOOD TRACKER

BEFORE	AFTER	THOUGHTS / NOTES ON YOUR MEDITATION
□ GOOD	□ GOOD	
□ NEUTRAL	□ NEUTRAL	
□ STRESSED	□ STRESSED	

SLEEP TRACKER

SLEEP QUALITY	HOW MANY HOURS DID YOU SLEEP?	DREAM NOTES
□ GOOD		
□ NEUTRAL	**WHAT TIME DID YOU GO TO BED?**	
□ STRESSED	□ AM □ PM	

SELF CARE TRACKER

MIND / SPIRIT	EXERCISE / PHYSICAL ACTIVITY

MINDFULNESS

POSITIVE AFFIRMATIONS	GRATITUDE

MEDITATION LOG

DATE		TIME		HOW LONG	

MOOD TRACKER

BEFORE	AFTER	THOUGHTS / NOTES ON YOUR MEDITATION
□ GOOD	□ GOOD	
□ NEUTRAL	□ NEUTRAL	
□ STRESSED	□ STRESSED	

SLEEP TRACKER

SLEEP QUALITY	HOW MANY HOURS DID YOU SLEEP?	DREAM NOTES
□ GOOD		
□ NEUTRAL	WHAT TIME DID YOU GO TO BED?	
□ STRESSED	□ AM □ PM	

SELF CARE TRACKER

MIND / SPIRIT	EXERCISE / PHYSICAL ACTIVITY

MINDFULNESS

POSITIVE AFFIRMATIONS	GRATITUDE

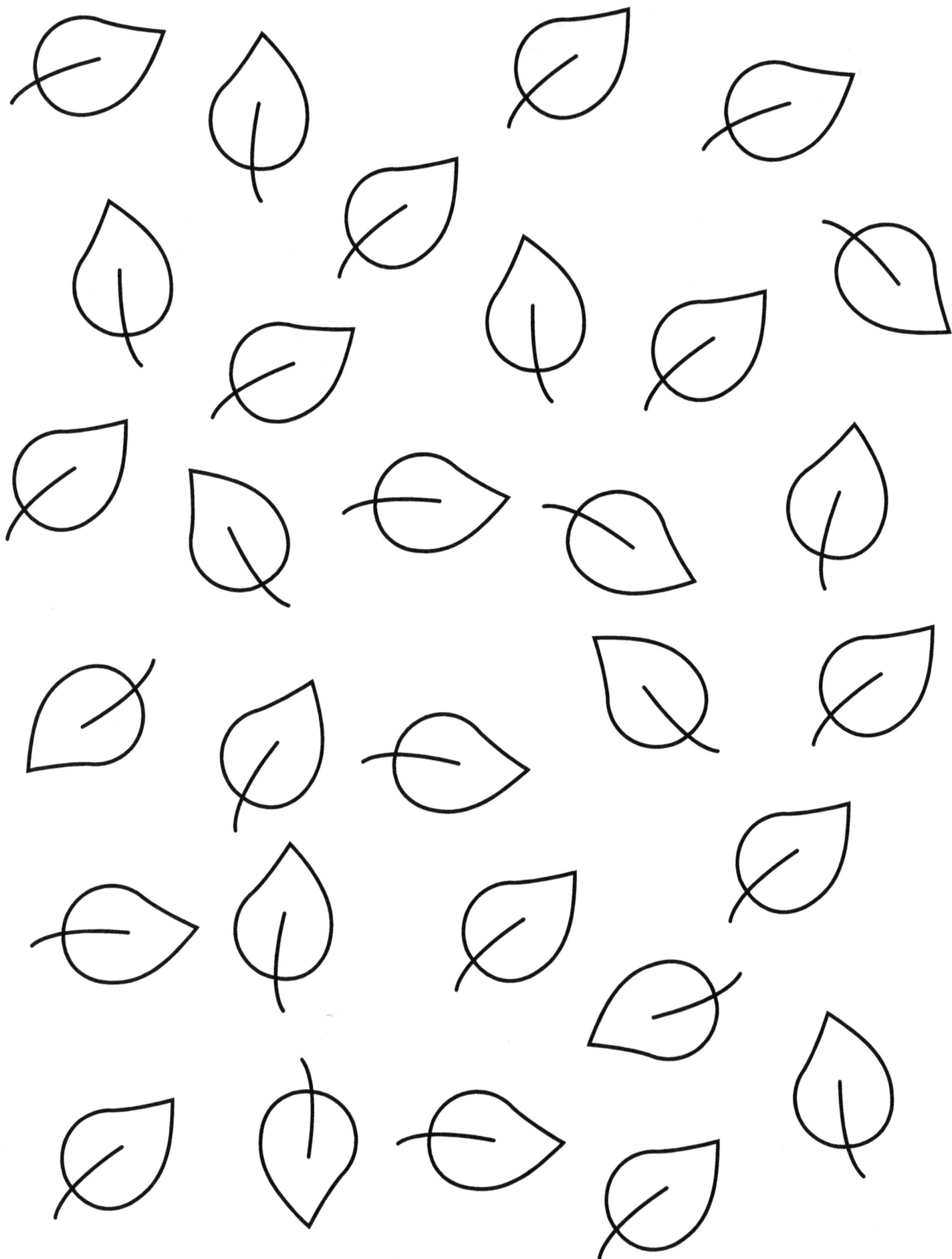